WADE RYANN

JUST MOVE

Finding happiness in exercise and knowing the benefits it brings.

INTRODUCTION

L et wisdom inspire you to get moving.
still, you might have observed how the benefits of exercising carry over into day-to-day life, If you're someone who works out regularly. Yoga, for illustration, can educate us to take deep breaths in stressful situations. From dancing, we learn that a good mood can be contagious. And a hard cardio session tells us that a fast heartbeat isn't always a sign of fear.

And that's not all a single good drill can incontinently change your mood, make you feel stronger and further confident, and bring you near to the people you exercise with. The internal health benefits of exercise are inarguable, and they apply whether your preferred physical exertion is running, toning, or swimming; whether you're an amateur or a pro athlete.

This book will exfoliate light on how and why physical exertion affects your mood, your sense of purpose, and your tone- perception – and show you that movement is a crucial factor in mortal happiness. By the end, you'll have all the more reason and alleviation to get moving.

Get to know

what's really behind the " runner's high ";
    why people get addicted to exercise; and
    how a hard drill can change your perspective on life.

Exercise can unnaturally change our perception of ourselves and also Green exercise.

At Tough Mudder, a periodic handicap marathon that now happens all over the world, actors face intimidating physical obstacles with names similar to " Arctic Enema, " " Boa Constrictor, " or " Graduation to Hell. " For the final handicap on the course, " Electroshock remedy, " actors have to run through curtains of cables galvanized with over,000 volts.

Why you might ask yourself, would anyone subdue themselves to similar torture? We've all heard that exercise is good for us — how it strengthens our hearts and lungs and helps us help conditions like diabetes. That's why so numerous of us like to make New Year's judgments to move more, knowing it'll make us healthier and live longer. But numerous people don't know about the other important benefits of exercise — how it can help us find happiness, stopgap, connection, and courage.

Around the world, people who are physically active are happier and further satisfied with their lives. They have a stronger sense of purpose and experience more gratefulness, love, and stopgap. They feel more connected to their communities and are less likely to suffer from loneliness or come depressed. These benefits are seen throughout the lifetime, including among those living with serious internal and physical health challenges. That's true whether their favored exertion is walking, running, swimming, dancing, biking, playing sports, lifting weights, or rehearsing yoga.

Why is movement linked to such a wide range of cerebral benefits? One reason is its important and profound good on the brain. Then are five surprising ways that being active is good for your brain and how you can harness these benefits yourself.

1. The exercise " high " primes you to connect with others

Although generally described as a runner's high, an exercise-convinced mood boost isn't exclusive to running. An analogous bliss can be set up in any sustained physical exertion.

Scientists have long suspected that endorphins are behind the high, but exploration shows the high is linked to another class of brain chemicals endocannabinoids(the same chemicals mimicked by cannabis) — what neuroscientists describe as " don't worry, be happy " chemicals.

Areas of the brain that regulate the stress response, including the amygdala and prefrontal cortex, are rich in receptors for endocannabinoids. When endocannabinoid motes lock into these receptors, they reduce anxiety and induce a state of pleasure. Endocannabinoids also increase dopamine in the brain's price system, which further energies passions of sanguinity.

This exercise high also primes us to connect with others, by adding the pleasure we decide from being around other people, which can strengthen connections. numerous people use exercise as an occasion to connect with musketeers or loved bones

. Among wedded couples, when consorts exercise together, both mates report further closeness latterly that day, including feeling loved and sup- ported.

Another study set up that on days when people exercise, they report more positive relations with musketeers and family. As one runner said to me, " My family will occasionally shoot me out running, as they know that I'll come back a much better person. "

2. Exercise can make your brain more sensitive to joy

When you exercise, you give a low-cure jolt to the brain's price centers the system of the brain that helps you anticipate pleasure, feel motivated, and maintain a stopgap. Over time, regular exercise remodels the price system, leading to advanced circulating situations of dopamine and more available dopamine receptors. In this way, exercise can both relieve depression and expand your capacity for joy.

These changes can also repair the neurological annihilation extorted by substance abuse. Substance abuse lowers the position of dopamine in your brain and reduces the vacuity of dopamine receptors in the price system. As result, people floundering with dependence can feel unmotivated, depressed, asocial, and unfit to enjoy ordinary pleasures. Exercise can reverse this.

Well, facing our fears by prostrating physical challenges can fully transfigure our understanding of what we're able of – and come as a tremendous source of commission. The tone- stated thing of the people who come up with the Tough Mudder obstacles isn't to torture people, but to produce challenges that encourage them to overcome common phobias – of height, cold, confined spaces – and give them a sense of confidence, frippery, and community.

Psychologically, the key to transubstantiating fear into courage seems to be giving subjects an element of control. When rats are shocked by a researcher with no control over when or for how long the shocks are delivered, they come helpless, traumatized, and depressed. But when they're given the capability to turn off the shocks by turning a wheel, they bravely learn to do so – and come more flexible to future stress in the process.

also, humans grow with their challenges. DPI Adaptive Fitness in Fairfax, Virginia, is a spa specializing in training those with physical constraints or disabilities. When trainees first come by, their coach encourages them to set themselves a thing so high that numerous believe they will noway achieve it. For illustration, when Joana Bonilla first arrived at DPI, she had just lost the use of her legs due to the autoimmune complaint lupus. She allowed

she'd noway be suitable to drive again. With her coach, she set the thing of being suitable to throw 100 punches in 30 seconds, which would help her develop enough upper body strength to heave herself from her wheelchair into an auto. After just three months of training, Joana was suitable to meet the thing, and just a few weeks later, she bought a new auto.

Since your body is constantly transferring feedback to your brain, learning an uncomfortable, insolvable- evident physical challenge can literally transfigure your sense of tone. Performing an important feat, for illustration, sends a communication to your brain that you're important. In this way, exercise can challenge indeed our most deeply held beliefs about ourselves – as numerous DPI trainees can attest.

Also, " Green exercise " gates into the ancient mortal desire to connect with nature.

Exercising outside has numerous benefits for your body and mind.

exploration extensions acknowledge that physical exertion can help keep you healthy. sharing in regular physical exertion reduces blood pressure, and blood sugar situations and helps with maintaining a healthy weight. In addition, interacting with nature on a diurnal base has been shown to ameliorate internal health by reducing situations of stress, and anxiety and indeed perfecting symptoms of depression.

Green exercise, which is considered any physical exertion that takes place outdoors, has been shown to ameliorate both physical and internal health. Conditioning can be purposeful similar to visiting a neighborhood theater or riding a bike, incidental similar to interacting with people while walking to the grocery store or walking in the demesne, as well as circular like looking at trees through a window or viewing filmland of nature scenes. It includes a variety of conditioning similar as gardening, cycling, walking, steed riding, flying harpies, walking the canine, or sharing in a neighborhood design like planting flowers.

In one study, children endured out-of-door tutoring over regular intervals of one academy day per week in the timber. Their out-of-door - literacy program included chances to be physically active during free choice conditioning and through adult guided planned conditioning. As compared to children in a regular academy setting, " children in the out-of-door classes show advanced exertion situations than their peers in the academy erecting the intervention group in the outside have a statistically significant lesser decline of cortisol compared to the control group. " Cortisol is a hormone released in the body in response to stress. It triggers the flight or fight response as part of our mortal survival medium. It's advanced in the morning and smallest at night. When cortisol situations are lower, we're calmer.

Another study used an out-of-door Behavioral Health Care approach that combined traditional internal health comforting with nature gests for youth periods 18- 23 formerly diagnosed with internal health issues similar to mood diseases, substance abuse, and anxiety. Experimenters set up that actors who completed the program had a reduction in symptoms of torture and interpersonal difficulties and an increased sense of purpose while sharing in the intervention. These benefits continued after discharge.

Now that you've learned about the multitudinous positive goods that movement has on our internal health, would you like to know what's indeed better for your brain than exercise?

Exercising outdoors!

Nature has the power to fill us with wonder and admiration, give us a sense of belonging, and make us more alert. Combined with physical exertion, it has tremendous positive goods on our internal health. For illustration, within just five twinkles of " green exercise," as it's occasionally called, people report major positive changes in their mood and outlook.

still, just a flashback that the mortal brain evolved over a long period of time, the utmost of which humans spent outside running, If you're wondering why.

Indeed, brain reviews show that our dereliction brain state is different outside than it's outdoors. Outdoors, where Americans now spend an average of 93 percent of their time, our dereliction state shows activation in the brain areas responsible for memory, language, and social commerce, and slightly leans toward negativity – which is why we're more likely to engage in reflection, tone- review, or worry indoors.

But when we're in nature, our dereliction brain state more nearly resembles the calm, disentangled state achieved by educated meditators. We witness lower anxiety, are more apprehensive of our surroundings, and slip into a state experimenters call soft seductiveness.

Psychologist Alexandra Rosati believes that these two different countries of the mortal brain – indoors and outside, ruminating and aware – correspond to two different types of cognition that were pivotal to our ancestors' survival. The ruminating state is the outgrowth of the elaboration of social cognition, our capability to suppose about other people and cooperate within small groups. The aware state derives from rustling cognition, our capability to be alert when hunting and gathering food. Naturally, the ultimate is brought out stylishly when we're outside.

People who feel connected to nature tend to spend further time in this rustling condition, and maybe, as a consequence, experience lesser life satisfaction, purpose, and happiness. They're also less likely to be depressed and anxious.

The Green Gym action in the UK makes use of the joy we decide from movement and nature by transferring levies to do nature-grounded conditioning with a social focus, similar to planting community auditoriums. Experimenters at the University of Westminster showed that after eight weeks of the program, Green Gym levies showed a 20 percent increase in their cortisol awakening response – the hormonal boost that gets us up and going in the morning, and which is frequently suppressed in depressed people. In conclusion, if you're working on maintaining or perfecting your health by including physical exertion, consider going outdoors as part of your routine so you can boost both your physical and internal health.

The high we witness from physical exertion is an ancient medium helping us persist, thrive, and fraternize

High-intensity exercises are the rearmost trend in fitness. But what does that actually mean? Exercising to the point of complete muscle fatigue or until you throw up? Or a commodity a little less violent, but hard enough that you can not talk.

One of the most important rudiments is the intensity of your drill, so it's important to get it right. While the utmost guidelines recommend moderate-intensity exercise most days of the week, working at a high intensity can help you burn further calories, save time with shorter exercises, and increase your fitness position.

As early as 1885, Scottish champion Alexander Bain described what we now call the " runner's high " the feeling of bliss and intoxication that sets in after a prolonged period of jogging. Bain likened this high to a spiritual experience, but others have compared it to being in love, and the goods of all kinds of mind-altering medicines.

Curiously, from a neurological viewpoint, the medicine that the runner's high comes closest to is cannabis. Recent studies have shown that the long run greatly increases situations of endocannabinoids in our brains. These are a class of chemicals, and cannabis mimics their goods of them on the brain. Endocannabinoids are known for lessening pain, boosting mood, and driving fresh sense-good chemicals and neurotransmitters similar to dopamine and endorphins. When you start out on your run, your body goes through a transition Your breathing may come heavy, and you might notice your palpitation quicken as the heart pumps harder to move oxygenated blood to your muscles and brain.

As you hit your stride, your body releases hormones called endorphins. Popular culture identifies these as the chemicals behind " runner's high, " a short- continuing, deeply ecstatic state following violent exercise. checks have revealed runner's high to be rather rare, still, with a maturity of athletes noway passing it. Indeed, numerous distance runners feel simply drained or indeed revolted at the end of a long race, not joyful,

And though endorphins help muscles from feeling pain, it's doubtful that endorphins in the blood contribute to an ecstatic feeling or any mood change at all. exploration shows that endorphins don't pass the blood-brain hedge.

That relaxed post-run feeling may rather be due to endocannabinoids — biochemical substances analogous to cannabis but naturally produced by the body.

Exercise increases the situation of endocannabinoids in the bloodstream, Linden explains. Unlike endorphins, endocannabinoids can move fluently through the cellular hedge separating the bloodstream from the brain, where these mood-perfecting neuromodulators promote short-term psychoactive goods similar to reduced anxiety and passion for calm.

Endocannabinoids also help cover us against anxiety and depression. The internal benefits don't stop when you finish your run — regular cardiovascular exercise can spark the growth of new blood vessels to nourish the brain. Exercise may also produce new brain cells in certain locales through a process called neurogenesis, which may lead to an overall enhancement in brain performance and help cognitive decline.

" Exercise has a dramatic way to prevent depression ". " It blunts the brain's response to physical and emotional stress. "

What's more, the hippocampus — the part of the brain associated with memory and literacy — has been set up to increase in volume in the smarts of regular trampolinists. Other internal benefits include

bettered working memory and concentrate
   More task-switching capability
   Elevated mood
   By making running or jogging(or any aerobic exercise) a regular part of your routine, you stand to earn further than just physical earnings over time. Voluntary exercise is the single stylish thing one can do to decelerate the cognitive decline that accompanies normal aging.
   The weight-loss medicine Rimonabant, for illustration, was designed to suppress appetite by blocking endocannabinoid receptors. rather, it brought about dramatic increases in anxiety and depression in clinical trials, indeed leading to four self-murders, and was permanently banned. Again, one recent study showed that just 30 twinkles of exercise can make people vulnerable to severe anxiety convinced by the medicine CCK- 4. In this study, the effect of exercise was original to taking an opiate-like Ativan.

And that's not all endocannabinoids also make us more social. In one trial conducted by experimenters at the Sapienza University of Rome, people who exercised for 30 twinkles before playing a social game were much more generous and collaborative than people who didn't. an enterprise like GoodGym in London harnesses the social energy generated by physical exertion they organize collaborative runs that shoot levies to do all feathers of social systems in their communities, similar to visiting socially insulated senior people.

Luckily for those of us who'd rather eat a broom than run a stage around the block, the runner's high isn't confined to running. It's proven to appear after all kinds of relatively exhausting physical exertion that takes further than 20 twinkles, whether that's swimming, cycling, or speed-walking. therefore, the explosion of brain chemicals from prolonged exercise might be more directly called a " continuity high. " Why would our smarts make us feel so good about exhausting our bodies? The rearmost proposition traces this miracle back to our foremost ancestors. Continuity high likely evolved to keep us hunting and gathering for long ages of time, making us more likely to find food and survive. And the increased amenability to cooperate and partake after physical exertion could also have had an evolutionary benefit it made nimrods more likely to partake in their pillages with the lineage.

The mortal brain can get hooked on exercise in a way that resembles a medicine dependence – but with much more positive issues.

What causes exercise dependence?

Exercise releases endorphins and dopamine. These are the same neurotransmitters released during medicine use. An exercise addict feels pride and joy when exercising. When they stop exercising, the neurotransmitters go down. An addict has to exercise further to spark the chemical release.

Exercise dependence generally starts with a desire for physical fitness. An eating complaint, similar to anorexia nervosa or bulimia, may lead to an unhealthy preoccupation with exercise. A body dysmorphic complaint, or body image complaint, may also beget exercise dependence.

Who's at threat of exercise dependence?

People who feel pressure to stay in shape are at threat of developing exercise dependence. And people who are fat and set out on an extreme weight loss authority may also be at threat of exercise dependence.

Experimenters at the University of Southern CaliforniaTrusted Source presume that 15 percent of exercise addicts are also addicted to cigarettes, alcohol, or lawless medicines. An estimated 25 percent may have other dependencies, similar to coitus dependence or shopping dependence.

In some cases, former medicine addicts and alcohol abusers turn to exercise to fill the void left by once dependents. This is analogous to the way a smoker may come addicted to caffeine after quitting cigarettes. Experts suppose regular physical exertion can act as a healthy stage- heft for addicting substances. That's because exercise and medicines of abuse work on the analogous corridor of your brain. They both spark your price pathway, which triggers the release of sense-good chemicals like serotonin and dopamine.

We need further exploration to know exactly how exercise affects dependence. But studies show it might

Ease pullout. Regular exercise can lessen anxiety, depression, and stress. These are common symptoms you might get during recovery that can lead to relapse.

you can get a really strong appetite to use medicines when you try to avoid them. Exercise can distract you from jones

or make them less important.

Replace your triggers. A new exercise routine can give you a commodity to do and make your social network. This might help you avoid people, places, or effects that remind you of medicines.

Help you suppose easily. Regular physical exertion can help your mind work more. Your odds of relapse might go down when your studies are more stable.

Ameliorate your sleep.However, it's common to get wakefulness when you try to avoid medicines or alcohol If you have SUD. Regular exercise might help you fall asleep briskly and get better quality rest at night.

Boost your tone- regard and tone- control. It's easier to manage stressful stuff when you feel good about yourself.

Exercises That Can Help

Early exploration shows aerobic exercise and resistance training might help with dependence recovery. But right now, there's not enough substantiation to say that one kind of physical exertion is better than another. unborn studies should help us learn more.

Aerobic, or cardio, exercises get your heart rate over for a sustained period. That includes

Walking
Running
Swimming
Boxing
Hiking
Light gardening
Dancing
Water calisthenics
Resistance, or strength- training, exercises work your muscles. exemplifications include

Some kinds of yoga
Toning
Push-ups or sit-ups
syllables or lunges
Heavy gardening, is similar to digging.
When experimenters first started studying the miracle of " exercise dependence " in the late 1960s, they ran into a big problem. No matter how important plutocrats they offered, they couldn't find any regular trampolinists willing to see what would be if they stopped exercising for a while. And if they did subscribe up, actors tended to cheat and lie, pretending they hadn't worked out when they had.

This yarn illustrates that the " continuity high " people get from abidance sports isn't the only way exercise can be likened to medicines. Because it activates our brain's price system in analogous ways to substances like cocaine and heroin – stimulating the release of sense-good chemicals like endocannabinoids, dopamine, endorphins, and noradrenaline – regular physical exertion can be just as addicting as those substances.

For tone-described exercise junkies, for illustration, missing a single drill can increase anxiety and perversity. And after several missed exercises, numerous of them report signs of depression and wakefulness. They also show the same attentional bias as other addicts when shown images of people working out, the brain of an exercise null fires up in the same way as when you show cigarettes to a smoker.

still, there are some important ways in which exercise dependence differs from other habit-forming dependencies. First of all, it takes our brain longer to get hooked on exercise than on medicines, because the chemical changes that physical exertion effect in our brain are less violent and more sluggish.

For illustration, mice who are made to exercise each day for two weeks don't show symptoms of exercise dependence latterly. But after six weeks, a commodity in their brain seems to flip, and indeed with no bone

forcing or awarding them, they can hardly stop running. analogous studies on humans show that we tend to get hooked on exercise after exercising four times a week for six weeks.

As with other medicines, regularly getting " high " on physical exertion sluggishly changes the chemical structure of your brain. But the great thing is that rather than making you less sensitive to its positive goods, as happens with chemical medicines, regular exercise makes you more sensitive to them. This happens because exercise increases the receptors for endocannabinoids in your brain and makes dopamine cells more responsive. This is why, in stark discrepancy to medicines, the further exercise you do, the better you feel about it.

Humans are hardwired to decide pleasure from accompanied by physical exertion.

Fitness trends come and go, but if you observe them nearly, you'll discover that numerous recent exercise modes partake in an analogous format that supercharges a formerly being exertion by adding accompanied movement and community spirit.

Consider Tae Bo, for illustration, which adds rudiments of cotillion choreography to boxing, or SoulCycling, which brings a social, nearly spiritual, element to the lone sport of inner cycling.

Since the morning of history, humans have gathered to move together. First, in all kinds of social, idolater, or religious rituals; currently, in group exercise classes. As anthropologists have observed all over the world, moving in accord seems to make people feel more connected – to each other, but also to commodities bigger than themselves. French sociologist Émile Durkheim called the joyous tone- preponderancy humans can decide from moving together " collaborative effervescence. "

Coincidence seems to be a crucial factor in producing similar collaborative joy. In fact, coinciding physical exertion with others seems to be an ancient mortal kickback. When we feel close to a person, for illustration, our breathing, jiffs, and indeed brain exertion tend to automatically align themselves. And we're actually more at coinciding with another person's slightly irregular beat than with a perfect computer-generated meter.

The reason why this has such an important effect on our psyche can be explained through a process called proprioception, by which our brain senses what our body is doing in space. When we move, our body is constantly transferring feedback to our brain about the movement. And when we see others performing the same movements that we feel ourselves doing, our brain assimilates these sensations into a veritably satisfying perception of oneness. As your fellow humans begin to feel like a part of yourself, you also come more likely to partake and cooperate with them.

The related effect of moving in coincidence can be demonstrated in babies as youthful as fourteen months old. One study showed that babies are more likely to help a foreigner pick up dropped pencils after they had bounced to music in sync with that person.

Transcending our individual limitations and adding collective trust feel to be the main functions of accompanied movement, and it's presumably why humans employ it in so numerous social, religious, or military rituals. Whether it's a huntsman-gatherer lineage performing a cotillion ritual or council scholars in a pilates class, accompanied movement helps us leave our self-esteem before and bond with people we aren't related to.

Music is also a performance-enhancing medicine.

Some exercise scientists could convincingly argue that when Ethiopian Haile Gebrselassie broke the world record in the 2000 cadence race during a US running competition in 1998, he was actually on performance-enhancing medicine. before that day, Gebrselassie had managed to move event organizers to play the pop song " Scatman " during the race – one of his favorite songs, and the song he'd trained to. When he heard the familiar upbeat airplay over the giant colosseum speakers, Gebrselassie was suitable to run faster than he ever had ahead.

The power of music to push us beyond our physical limits can hardly be exaggerated. Musicologists have long described music as ergogenic, or work-enhancing, and wisdom is chancing further and further substantiation to back up this claim. One recent study set up that people who hear to music during their exercises consume lower oxygen than those who don't. And indeed cases with high blood pressure last 51 seconds longer during a cardiovascular stress test when they're allowed to run on the routine to their favorite melodies.

Costas Karageorghis has made a career out of the performance-enhancing powers of music his job is to curate drill playlists for some of the world's stylish athletes. A trained sports psychologist, explains that the stylish drill songs generally have a strong, energetic beat, a tempo of 120 to 140 beats per nanosecond, and motivational lyrics that include words similar as " work, " " go, " or " run. " Eminem's " Till I Collapse, " for case, estimated to be the most popular drill song of all time, ticks nearly all of these boxes.

similar positive, familiar songs have the power to deliver us a redundant burst of sense-good chemicals like adrenaline, dopamine, and endorphins during our drill. Upbeat warbles and inspirational lyrics can also help us frame physical discomfort more positively.

Humans ' deep-seated appetite to move to music has indeed led to medical cautions. notorious neurologist Oliver Sacks liked to tell the story of a woman whose leg was paralyzed after a complex bone fracture. Croakers believed that the communication between her leg muscles and her spinal cord had been cut fully, yet when she heard her favorite Irish ploy, her bottom spontaneously started tapping. penetrating muscle memory with music remedy, the woman learned to walk again.

Enduring physical rigors trains internal strength.

Pain is insolvable to ignore — as soon as we feel commodity hurt we're wired to start allowing it to help unborn injuries And, occasionally, discomfort is indeed a sign you need to back off. But utmost of the time, with proper form and the applicable exertion, exercise-convinced pain is really just a sign of cardiovascular exertion or muscle breaking down and erecting back stronger heads. Discomfort can gesture " time to decelerate down, " " time to horrify, " or " time to push on indeed harder " — and what your body is trying to communicate is nearly entirely dependent on what you want to hear.

In any kind of athletic performance, it's ineluctable you're going to face discomfort, physical or emotional. But it's your perception of and response to it that will determine how important power it has over your performance.

Powering through that healthy discomfort isn't just the avenue to getting fitter and faster it also helps you understand your physical limits more directly so it hurts a little lower coming time.

But how do you tune out the blubbering and tune into the winning? Then are some proven strategies to concentrate less on the pain and further on learning your factual limits.

1. Develop an awareness practice

Doing any of these strategies(let alone all of them) requires a position of moxie and familiarity with the body, so you can distinguish true discomfort from factual pain, which could be motioning an injury.

The most effective and effective way to do this is awareness training. awareness requires trouble outside the spa, but putting in the time comes with serious nets, including better pain control, also bettered sleep, bettered provocation, and lower stress.

2. Plan for and embrace discomfort

Any kind of particular stylish performance will involve discomfort because you're pushing yourself past what you've done ahead. " awaiting discomfort allows us to accept and indeed embrace it as a sign that effects are going right rather than effects are going awry. "

Going into a drill or race, suppose about the moves ahead of you and how your body has replied in the past. However, anticipate the cramping as soon as you start your ascent If you always get side aches sprinting uphill. However, anticipate wanting to throw up and cry contemporaneously, If the moment's WOD involves burpee box jumps. when we accept the discomfort, two really important effects be First, we can devote our headpiece to negotiating the physical task at hand — setting the pace and breathing, rather than fighting the uncomfortable passions. Second, we avoid piling redundant pain on top of judgment(" If I were fit, I wouldn't be feeling this. "), fussing about it(" If I feel like this formerly, there's no way I 'm going to be suitable to finish. "), or catastrophizing it(" If I feel like this now I might as well quit because I 'm not going to get the results I want. ").

3. suppose pain as power

Pain is incontestably a negative sensation, right? Actually, it's allowing it as negative that makes it so. Every feeling that comes into your body on the field, during a race, or in the spa is fully neutral until we fix a positive or negative marker to them. Rapid twinkle, muscle pressure, and contending studies could be either excitement or anxiety — but which you choose to believe you're feeling will directly affect your performance. When we're in a positive emotional frame, we're likely to perform better.

Get your mind right As fatigue or pain starts to submerge your body, suppose of this new sensation as a flood tide of strength and energy rather. Feel the vigor coursing through your blood sluice, and shoot the sensation where you need it most — focus on a sluice of strength and power moving through your muscles, amping your closes for the long hauls left, or powering your shoulders for one further press. Allowing discomfort this way makes you more likely to embrace the feeling as opposed to avoiding it.

4. Set small pretensions

Take a race afar by afar, and take each WOD exercise by exercise. occasionally, when(the exertion) gets really tough, we just need to make it to the coming light pole or indeed the coming breath. When we resolve up the drill or competition to the coming little piece, the whole picture isn't gaping us down.

The strategy of setting small pretensions is a part distraction, part consolation from small triumphs When you feel like you're ready to drop but push yourself to churn out just one further rep, it instills the confidence that perhaps you in fact have a little further energy left despite your crying muscles. Breaking the drill into gobbets effectively teaches your brain that pain isn't the real index that you're done with. Plus, breaking down the race or drill into small pretensions helps the time move briskly — and, thus, helps dissipate the sensation of pain. generally, this tough time passes, and you'll be back at it in many twinkles.

5. Queue up a cue word

suppose about what you need most when you feel tired or uncomfortable — power, energy, focus, provocation — and make a list of words that elicit that feeling strongest to you. They can be as straightforward as action words or expressions like " explode, " " voyage, " " get after it, " or commodity tête-à-tête motivating to only you. " I 've had athletes use the name of their nonage practice field or their youth trainer to evoke passions of fun or enjoyment, ". When your drill becomes wearisome, reach for your cue word and put it on reprise until the meaning sinks in.

6. Breathe

Just by simply fastening your breath and controlling your respiratory rate, you can alter your heart rate, clear your mind, and achieve an optimal position of thrill. Not only will controlling your physiological response help dissipate the pain, but internal clarity will help you make smarter opinions on what you may need to acclimate in order to avoid discomfort. Plus, it takes your mind off of the painful sensations your body is passing and places it on another physical sensation that you can control. Whether you want to control or observe is over to you. Being with your breath, not trying to control, judge, or change it's one strategy. But feeling the coolness of air coming in and the warmth of it going out, noticing the rise and fall of the stomach can also be effective. There's no one

right way.

7. Distract yourself

Find a spot on the ground, sing a song in your head, count the number of colors around you — the mind can only concentrate on so important at any given time, so offer it commodity other than pain to obsess over. Another option Shift your focus to a part of your body that isn't in pain, like having loose and relaxed hands while running up a hill, enough any distraction works, except fastening on effects that are beyond your control, like another runner's time or rainfall conditions.

8. Observe the sensations

These ways all work well to deaden low to moderate situations of pain but we all have a threshold. When the pain of commodity becomes so great, you have no choice but to tune into the passions it elicits. However, your stylish bet is acceptance rather than resistance, If you pass the point of action. exploration shows that elite players are more comfortable defying discomfort, while amateur athletes use avoidance more.

Rather than freaking out, control what you can — breathing rate, running pace, muscle pressure — and suppose about " bringing intention " to your paining muscles. Physiologically, this gives further oxygen to those areas — energy overflows where attention goes. But indeed if you can't alleviate the pain, bringing mindfulness to a body part shines a flashlight on it — brings it to life in a certain way.

For Shawn Bearden, host of a popular podcast on ultrarunning, abidance sport was a way out of his depression. He explains that training his body to endure similar extreme physical difficulties is a way to cultivate internal strength that carries over to another corridor of his life. For illustration, during the race, Bearden tries to concentrate on the present moment and draws strength from allowing his favored bones

– chops that have also helped him manage his depression.

Abidance athletes like Bearden don't inescapably seek out their sport because they're extremely flexible, but because the sport trains them to come extremely flexible. In fact, histories of depression, dependence, and anxiety are common among the world's top ultrarunners.

In 2015, when experimenters followed athletes contending in the Yukon Arctic Ultra, they set up that the athletes ' capability to dogface on through extreme conditions was linked to veritably high situations of the hormone irisin. Irisin is best known for helping our bodies burn fat as energy, but it also stimulates the brain's price system, acting as a natural provocation- supporter and antidepressant. Irisin in the bloodstreams of sharing athletes was largely elevated before the marathon and climbed indeed advanced during it.

Irisin belongs to a class of proteins called myokines, which are manufactured by our muscles during physical exertion. Myokines are known to boost our physical and cognitive performance, palliate pain, reduce depression and inflammation, and indeed kill cancer cells. Because they can cover the brain from some of the neurodegenerative symptoms of conditions similar to depression and Parkinson's, scientists have started calling these salutary proteins " stopgap motes. "

Exercising at similar high intensity and volume as extreme abidance athletes can stimulate violent bursts of myokine release. But you don't need to be an ultrarunner to harness the positive powers of the stopgap motes. A single hour of biking is enough to release about 35 different myokines into your bloodstream.

As this book has hopefully shown, the myriad benefits of physical exertion are available to all of us. As humans, we're hardwired to find happiness in movement.

Conclusion

For humans, the benefits of exercise extend far beyond perfecting our physical health. Because of our evolutionary history as nimrods and gatherers, mortal smarts are hardwired to decide happiness, meaning, and a sense of belonging from physical exertion – especially if that physical exertion takes place to music, in nature, or alongside others. The numerous different brain chemicals released during exercise have been shown to reduce anxiety and depression, palliate the physical and internal symptoms of colorful ails, and make us more likely to trust and support each other.

practicable advice

Just move!

Still, let it get moving! No matter your age, or your fitness position, If you take down a single piece of alleviation from this book. However, why not plan a daily walk in the demesne? Or if walking isn't an option for you, shake it out to a good song once in a while, If sweating in the spa isn't for you.